THE ART OF HEALING

FROM INFIDELITY

STRATEGIES AND STEPS FOR

REBUILDING A STRONG AND

LOVING RELATIONSHIP AFTER

INFIDELITY

ROBERT .E. JAMES

TABLE OF CONTENTS

CHAPTER 1: UNDERSTANDING THE EFFECTS OF INFIDELITY ON RELATIONSHIPS

Infidelity is a very complex and emotionally charged issue that has the potential to destroy even the strongest of relationships. Infidelity may leave a path of broken hearts, destroyed trust, and psychological pain that typically persists long after the affair has ended. While the impact of infidelity differs per relationship or marriage, knowing its consequences is critical in navigating the perilous path of healing and rebuilding the relationship. While there is no one-size-fits-all explanation for why people cheat, current research reveals that a variety of psychological, social, and biological factors have a role. Individuals fall to the temptation of hidden affairs, sometimes driven by a lack of emotional fulfillment, sexual unhappiness, or a desire for novelty and excitement, which has serious ramifications for their personal relationships. The erosion of trust is one of the most immediate and significant consequences of infidelity. When one spouse discovers that their significant other has been unfaithful, the foundation of any healthy relationship is damaged. The betrayed partner may find it difficult to trust their partner's words and conduct, resulting in persistent doubt and suspicion, even in unrelated situations. The betrayed spouse may doubt their own judgment and experience a severe sense of betrayal, resulting in a loss of self-esteem and confidence. Furthermore, the emotional consequences of infidelity or adultery can be catastrophic. Anger, hurt, and feelings of inadequacy are prevalent in the betrayed partner, while remorse and humiliation frequently torment the unfaithful partner. The emotional rollercoaster that accompanies the act of infidelity can be overpowering, resulting in an intense and tumultuous relationship climate. As both partners strive to understand their feelings and make sense of the infidelity, communication breaks down and disputes intensify. Infidelity affects not only the individuals involved, but also various elements of their existence. The social ramifications, for example, can be enormous, as friends and family members may take sides or provide unwanted advice, complicating the healing process. Furthermore, if the couple has children, the damage spreads to them, and they may feel confused, abandoned, or blame themselves for their parents' marital problems. While the immediate aftermath of infidelity can be painful and upsetting, it is critical to recognize that healing and rebuilding are possible. Relationships can be saved and even strengthened with the devotion and effort of both partners. The road to rehabilitation, however, is not easy. It necessitates open and honest communication, a desire to address the underlying causes of infidelity, and a commitment to restore trust and intimacy. Seeking expert assistance, such as couples

therapy or individual counseling, can

aid with the healing process. Trained

therapists can help couples heal and

navigate the challenges of infidelity

by navigating the complicated

aspects of the situation. Couples can

use therapy to address the underlying

issues that lead to the infidelity and

strive towards a more meaningful

and connected relationship.

Rebuilding trust is an important part

of recovering from infidelity. To demonstrate remorse and commitment to change, the unfaithful partner must commit persistent acts. Transparent and open communication is essential because the betrayed partner requires reassurance and honesty in order to regain trust. This procedure needs time and patience since trust is not readily reestablished. Both partners must be willing to put in the effort and accept responsibility for their actions. Though it is a difficult path, forgiveness is a vital step towards healing. It entails letting go of anger, hurt, and resentment and figuring out how to go ahead. Forgiveness does not imply forgetting or tolerating the act of infidelity; rather, it is a deliberate decision to release the emotional load and make room for emotional recovery. It is a personal process that varies from person to person, and it may necessitate professional assistance to manage. Finally, adultery has a profound and far-reaching impact on a relationship. It creates scars that may never completely heal, but with dedication, work, and the correct assistance, couples may repair their relationships and find a new level of connection and trust. Addressing the underlying issues, regaining trust, and finding forgiveness inside oneself are all necessary. Both spouses must be patient, compassionate, and understanding on this path.

To summarize, anyone who has experienced or is presently navigating the aftermath of an affair must grasp the impact of infidelity on relationships. Infidelity destroys trust, diminishes emotional well-being, and has an impact on many facets of one's life. Healing and rebuilding are, however, achievable with the correct support and commitment from both parties. To face the underlying issues that lead to adultery, it takes time, effort, and a commitment to do so. Couples with infidelity have the opportunity to emerge stronger and more connected on the other side of adultery via therapy, open communication, and forgiveness.

CHAPTER 2: RECOGNIZING THE PAIN: DEALING WITH THE REALITY OF INFIDELITY.

Infidelity is a deeply upsetting event that shatters trust and tests the links of love and devotion in a partnership. The difficult journey of dealing with infidelity should not be taken lightly; rather, it should be met with understanding, self-reflection, and open communication. This essay goes into the many facets of infidelity, examining the emotional toll, underlying reasons, and opportunities for healing and progress.

1. Recognizing the Effects of Infidelity:

Physical or emotional infidelity has a significant influence on both parties. Individuals who have been deceived suffer extreme emotions such as shock, rage, betrayal, humiliation, and a severe erosion of trust. To begin the healing process, it is critical to identify and validate these emotions. Recognizing the suffering is the first step towards recognizing and dealing with the problem.

2. The Multifaceted Causes of Infidelity:

Infidelity rarely occurs in isolation. It is critical to investigate the underlying factors that may have contributed to a partner's decision to cheat. These causes can include emotional separation, relational discontent, personal insecurities, unresolved prior traumas, or a lack of efficient communication. Understanding these underlying difficulties can provide insights into the dynamics of the relationship and allow both couples to work towards a healthier, more meaningful future.

3. Honest and Open Communication:

Partner communication must be open, honest, and nonjudgmental in order to rebuild trust following infidelity. Both parties must be free to express their emotions, concerns, and fears without fear of repercussions. Accountability, remorse, and the impact on the relationship dialogues should be tackled with kindness and a sincere desire to learn and repair.

4. Seeking Professional Assistance:

Couples who seek advice from skilled specialists, such as therapists or counselors who specialize in infidelity, typically benefit. These unbiased specialists may encourage constructive discussions, assist in navigating the pain, and guide both parties towards identifying underlying issues that contributed to the adultery. Professional support can help you rebuild trust, understand each other's needs, and establish healthy limits.

Restoring Trust and Healing:

Rebuilding trust takes time and involves consistency, transparency, and, most crucially, consistency. The unfaithful partner must be willing to accept responsibility for their acts and seek to recover trust by behaviors that support their partner's healing process. The deceived person must also be willing to forgive and make room for healing. This process might be difficult, but it is possible to reestablish trust and foster a stronger connection with sincere efforts from both partners.

Individual Reflection and Development:

Infidelity can be a catalyst for personal development and self-reflection. Both spouses should take some time to reflect on their involvement in the relationship's demise. This approach enables individuals to confront their own concerns, vulnerabilities, and behavioral patterns, resulting in personal growth and a more resilient foundation for the partnership in the future.

The Next Step:

While infidelity can have long-term consequences in a relationship, it can also serve as a catalyst for positive transformation. Couples can emerge from this difficult experience stronger and more committed if they communicate openly, seek expert help, and make sincere efforts to rebuild trust. The healing process allows partners to reassess their values, gain a better understanding of each other, and nurture a restored sense of closeness and connection.

Conclusion:

Infidelity is surely an unpleasant and difficult fact to confront, but it does not spell the end of a partnership. Recognizing the sorrow, comprehending the underlying causes, and embracing honest communication can lead to both couples' healing and growth. Rebuilding trust requires time, patience, and effort, but it is possible to survive and thrive after infidelity with commitment and willingness from both partners.

CHAPTER 3: EMOTIONAL PROCESSING: DEALING WITH ANGER, BETRAYAL, AND HURT

Emotions have an important role in influencing our experiences and perceptions. When confronted with situations that cause anger, betrayal, or hurt, it is critical to appropriately handle these emotions. This essay will go into the depths of these emotions, investigating their origins, influence, and healthy processing mechanisms. Individuals can discover healing, personal growth, and the ability to go on by acknowledging and resolving these feelings.

1. Recognize Anger: Anger is a strong emotion that frequently occurs in response to betrayal, hurt, or disappointed expectations. It is critical to understand that rage is a normal human emotion that functions as a protective mechanism. Unresolved anger, on the other hand, can be destructive and harmful to

one's well-being. This section delves into the origins of rage, its physical and emotional expressions, and appropriate expression and management measures.

2. Coping with Betrayal: Betrayal can leave people feeling emotionally hurt, questioning their trust, and experiencing disbelief. Betrayed emotions necessitate honest analysis and acknowledgement of the grief. Understanding the reasons for the

betrayal, participating in open discussion, and establishing boundaries can all help to speed up the healing process. This section digs into the complexities of betrayal and, if wanted, discusses solutions for self-care, forgiveness, and rebuilding trust.

3. Navigating Hurt and Healing: Hurt is a powerful feeling that arises from traumatic events such as rejection, loss, or disappointment. The healing

process begins with identifying and validating the pain, allowing oneself to grieve, and getting help from loved ones or specialists. This section discusses the stages of healing, the value of self-compassion, and ways for fostering resilience and emotional well-being.

4. Constructively Expressing Emotions: Emotional processing includes finding appropriate channels for expression. This section looks at

healthy ways to express anger, such as forceful speech, journaling, and physical activity. It also looks into ways for dealing with betrayal and hurt, such as engaging in self-care activities, creative expression, and obtaining professional help when necessary.

5. Developing Emotional Resilience: Developing emotional resilience is critical in the face of rage, betrayal, and pain. This section looks at ways

to improve emotional resilience, such as practicing mindfulness, creating healthy coping mechanisms, and cultivating positive relationships. Individuals who cultivate emotional resilience can manage these difficult emotions with greater ease and find strength in adversity.

6. Seeking Support: Seeking support from trusted persons or professionals can be beneficial in efficiently processing emotions. This section

emphasizes the significance of reaching out to caring friends, family members, or support groups who can offer understanding, direction, and a safe environment for expression. It also emphasizes the benefits of therapy or counseling in dealing with difficult emotions and obtaining a better understanding of oneself.

7. Accepting Personal Growth: Dealing with emotions like anger, betrayal, and hurt provides an

opportunity for personal growth and transformation. This section looks at how people might use difficult situations to spur positive transformation. It promotes self-reflection, the identification of personal values, and the setting of goals in order to promote growth and resilience.

Conclusion: Emotional processing is an important aspect of our emotional well-being and personal growth.

Individuals who understand and acknowledge their anger, betrayal, and hurt can negotiate these difficult emotions with self-compassion, resilience, and healthy expression. Seeking help, practicing mindfulness, and embracing personal growth are all strategies that can promote healing and pave the path for a more full and meaningful existence. Remember that processing emotions is a journey, and each step closer to emotional well-being and a brighter

future.

CHAPTER 4: REBUILDING TRUST: STRATEGIES FOR RESTORING YOUR PARTNER'S CONFIDENCE

The backbone of any healthy and happy relationship is trust. When trust is shattered, whether via dishonesty, betrayal, or other hurtful activities, the link between partners can suffer greatly. Rebuilding trust is a difficult task that necessitates dedication, vulnerability, and successful techniques. This extensive article delves into the difficult process of regaining trust in your partner, offering helpful insights and ways to promote healing, growth, and a healthier connection.

1. Recognize the Breach of confidence: Recognizing and comprehending the degree of the breach is the first step towards restoring confidence. This segment promotes open conversation and honest introspection between

spouses. It delves into the emotions and consequences of the breach on both persons, emphasizing the need of accepting responsibility for one's conduct.

2. Transparency and Open Communication: Restoring trust requires partners to communicate in a transparent and open manner. This section looks at how to create a safe space for discourse, actively listen to each other's concerns, and express

emotions constructively. It emphasizes the importance of consistent, clear communication as a foundation for trust restoration.

3. Demonstrating Genuine Remorse and responsibilities: Demonstrating genuine remorse and accepting responsibilities for one's conduct is an important part of regaining trust. This section goes into methods for expressing remorse, such as genuine apologies, verbalizing comprehension

of the harm done, and accepting responsibility for one's actions. It also emphasizes the significance of consistency in acts that are consistent with rebuilding trust.

4. Restoring Trust Through Actions: When it comes to repairing trust, actions speak louder than words. This section delves into practical ways for exhibiting trustworthiness, such as honesty, consistency, and commitment follow-through. It

emphasizes the need of being dependable, maintaining limits, and being transparent in everyday interactions.

5. Patience and Time: It takes time and patience to rebuild trust. This section discusses the necessity of letting the healing process evolve organically, without rushing or putting pressure on oneself or one's spouse. It emphasizes the importance

of consistency and patience as trust is steadily restored.

6. Seeking Professional intervention: In some circumstances, rebuilding trust may necessitate the intervention of a professional. This section discusses the advantages of obtaining therapy or counseling to help you manage the difficulties of rebuilding trust. It emphasizes the importance of a qualified professional in fostering

conversation, offering assistance, and investigating underlying issues that may have contributed to the breakdown of trust.

7. Trust-Building Exercises and Activities: This section includes exercises and activities that might help you reestablish trust. It looks at actions like developing emotional intimacy, practicing active listening, and participating in trust-building exercises. These activities allow

partners to reconnect, rebuild emotional links, and develop a sense of safety and security.

8. Self-Care and Healing: Individuals must prioritize self-care and personal healing in order to rebuild trust. This section goes into self-care practices such as practicing self-compassion, setting boundaries, and getting help from loved ones or professionals. It emphasizes the importance of individuals healing and regaining

their own sense of security and self-worth before fully repairing trust.

9. Forgiveness and Moving Forward: Forgiveness is a critical element of the trust restoration process. This section delves into the notion of forgiveness, offering advice on when forgiveness is feasible and how to cultivate it. It emphasizes the need of letting go of animosity and committing to the partnership again.

Conclusion:

Rebuilding trust is a difficult but necessary road for couples dealing with the fallout after a breach. It necessitates open communication, transparency, real contrition, and regular activities aimed towards restoring trust. It is possible to regain confidence and forge a stronger, more robust relationship with patience, time, and a willingness to seek professional help if necessary.

Individuals can engage on a journey of healing, growth, and restoring trust by applying the tactics provided in this thorough essay, which can lead to a more fulfilling and secure partnership. Remember that trust is difficult to rebuild, but with devotion, understanding, and a shared commitment, the link between couples can grow stronger than ever.

CHAPTER 5: COMMUNICATION AND HEALING: EFFECTIVE TECHNIQUES FOR EXPRESSING AND ADDRESSING EMOTIONS

Communication is the lifeblood of every healthy relationship, creating the groundwork for comprehension, connection, and growth. Effective communication becomes even more important in times of hurt, emotional distress, or conflict for healing and restoring harmony. This in-depth study delves into the art of communication in the context of healing, offering useful insights about expressing and addressing feelings. Individuals can encourage understanding, strengthen emotional relationships, and pave the path for healing and personal growth by learning the skills indicated in this article.

1. The Power of Effective Communication: The ability to communicate effectively is essential

for resolving problems, establishing emotional connection, and fostering a healthy relationship. This section discusses the importance of effective communication in the healing process, emphasizing its potential to decrease misconceptions, increase trust, and create a safe and supportive environment for expressing feelings.

2. Active Listening: Effective communication requires active

listening. This section looks into the fundamentals of active listening, such as paying full attention, using verbal and nonverbal clues, and reflecting back what has been heard. It offers practical advice on how to perfect active listening skills such as keeping eye contact, paraphrasing, and refraining from passing judgment. Individuals can foster an atmosphere of understanding and validation by being truly present and actively listening, allowing for healing and resolution.

3. Empathy and Validation: Empathy and validation are required for expressing and treating feelings. This section discusses the significance of empathy, which entails putting oneself in the shoes of another person and attempting to understand their emotions and point of view. It also emphasizes the importance of validation, which acknowledges the

other person's feelings as legitimate and deserving of attention. Individuals can establish a helpful environment for recovery by discussing strategies for generating empathy and providing validation.

Nonviolent Communication (NVC) is a strong strategy for resolving feelings and situations in a compassionate and non-confrontational manner. This section explains NVC in detail, including its ideas and practices. It examines the four NVC phases - observation, feeling, wants, and requests - and trains individuals in efficiently utilizing these procedures to express and treat their feelings. Individuals can encourage understanding, empathy, and resolution through NVC.

5. Constructive Expression of Negative Emotions:

Negative emotions like anger, bitterness, and sadness are a normal part of the healing process. However, properly expressing these emotions is critical for good communication. This section looks at ways to express unpleasant emotions in a healthy and non-destructive way. It emphasizes the necessity of adopting "I" expressions, avoiding blaming and criticism, and expressing wants and desires rather than ruminating on past wrongs. Individuals can make room for understanding and resolution by skillfully expressing negative feelings.

6. Conflict Resolution: While conflict is unavoidable in each relationship, it may be changed into an opportunity for growth and understanding. This section goes into effective conflict resolution tactics such as active listening, establishing common ground, and pursuing win-win solutions. It delves into the significance of assertiveness,

compromise, and respect during the resolution process. Individuals can address underlying difficulties, discover common ground, and forge a stronger connection by mastering conflict resolution skills.

7. Obtaining Professional Help: In some circumstances, obtaining professional help might help with successful communication and healing. This section delves into the function of therapists or counselors

in promoting conversation, providing guidance, and assisting persons in their recovery journey. It goes over the advantages of receiving professional assistance, such as acquiring fresh perspectives, developing communication strategies, and navigating deeper emotional concerns.

8. Develop Emotional Intelligence: Emotional intelligence is essential for effective communication and healing.

This section delves into the concept of emotional intelligence, which entails recognizing and comprehending one's own emotions as well as the emotions of others, and then using that understanding to drive communication. It teaches techniques for improving emotional intelligence, such as self-awareness, emotion management, and empathy. Individuals who cultivate emotional intelligence can communicate more effectively, address feelings with clarity and compassion, and deepen emotional ties.

9. Prioritizing Self-Care: Effective communication and healing necessitate prioritizing self-care. This section discusses the significance of self-care in the context of communication, emphasizing tactics such as setting boundaries, practicing self-compassion, and participating in activities that enhance emotional

well-being. Individuals who take care of themselves can approach conversation with strength and authenticity.

10. Developing a Growth mentality: A growth mentality is necessary for effective communication and healing. This section delves into the concept of a growth mindset, which entails accepting obstacles, viewing failures as chances for growth, and persevering in the face of adversity. It

emphasizes the importance of a growth mindset in developing resilience, encouraging open-mindedness, and supporting effective communication and healing.

Communication is a significant tool in the healing process because it allows people to express and confront their feelings, resolve problems, and build understanding and connection. Individuals can establish a supportive and loving atmosphere for healing and personal growth by practicing effective communication strategies such as active listening, empathy, nonviolent communication, and conflict resolution. It is critical to prioritize self-care, seek professional help when necessary, and develop emotional intelligence and a growth attitude. Individuals who use these tactics can handle difficult emotions and conflicts, create understanding and connection, and open the path for healing, growth, and deeper relationships. Remember that good communication takes time, practice, and a genuine desire for growth and understanding.

CHAPTER 6: RESTORING INTIMACY: FINDING EMOTIONAL AND PHYSICAL CONNECTION

Any effective and fulfilling relationship is built on intimacy. It forges a profound tie between two people that extends beyond the physical realm to include emotional, intellectual, and spiritual connections. Maintaining closeness, on the other hand, needs effort and attention, as challenges and life circumstances can often lead to a slow degradation of connection. But don't worry, it's always possible to rekindle closeness and rediscover the emotional and physical connection that once existed with commitment and understanding.

Recognizing the underlying causes that may have contributed to the fall of intimacy is the first step towards its restoration. A hectic lifestyle, professional pressures, family duties, and relationship difficulties are all common contributors. External events such as illness or financial difficulties may also play a role in some cases. By recognizing these aspects, both partners can obtain a greater knowledge of the issues they experience and the areas that need to be addressed.

Communication is essential for reestablishing connection. Couples can share their thoughts, problems, and desires without fear of being judged or defensive. Active listening is essential during these conversations because it demonstrates respect for each other's points of view and validates their emotions. Couples can get insight into each other's needs and work together to discover solutions that please both parties by actively listening.

Reestablishing emotional connection necessitates vulnerability and trust. It is critical to provide a safe atmosphere in which both partners may express their true self. This can be accomplished by scheduling regular check-ins during which each member can communicate their ideas and emotions without interruptions or distractions. Couples might identify prior injuries, misunderstandings, or unsolved problems that may have led to the estrangement through these interactions. Understanding the underlying causes enables healing and growth.

Furthermore, empathy is critical in reestablishing emotional intimacy. It entails being able to comprehend and share each other's emotions, resulting in a sense of connection and affirmation. Couples can strengthen their emotional bonds and gain a better knowledge of each other by actively empathizing with their partner's experiences.

Physical intimacy is an important aspect of every healthy relationship. However, it is frequently influenced by the emotional detachment that happens over time. It is critical to prioritize and create time for physical intimacy as an essential aspect of the relationship in order to restore it. This can include attempting new hobbies together or having intimate chats while cuddling to find new ways to connect physically. It is vital to remember that physical intimacy encompasses non-sexual contact, affection, and proximity in addition to sexual behaviors. Couples can reestablish their physical connection and rekindle any lost sparks by focusing on these factors.

In order to rebuild intimacy, you must make an effort to reconnect on a daily basis. Kindness, admiration, and compassion can go a long way towards developing intimacy. This can involve expressing gratitude to one another, surprising one another with modest gestures, or participating in activities that bring joy and laughter into the relationship. These acts of love not only build the emotional and physical bond, but also remind each partner of their worth and significance in the relationship.

Finally, obtaining professional assistance might be advantageous in the process of re-establishing closeness. Couples counseling or therapy provides a neutral and supportive atmosphere in which both spouses can work through their concerns and establish effective communication methods. A qualified therapist can provide direction and techniques to assist couples in healing, rebuilding trust, and rekindling intimacy

Rebuilding intimacy in a relationship takes time, effort, and open communication between partners. Here are some things you can take to rekindle your relationship's intimacy:

1. Consider the underlying issues: Take a time to consider the causes that may have contributed to the decline in intimacy. Determine whether there are any unsolved

disputes, prior injuries, or misconceptions that may be contributing to the estrangement.

2. Communicate clearly and truthfully: Make a safe space for both partners to share their thoughts, feelings, desires, and worries without fear of being judged or defensive. Active listening is used to comprehend each other's points of view and to validate each other's emotions.

3. Reestablish emotional connection: Share your vulnerabilities and worries with each other to foster a deeper emotional connection. Express thankfulness and appreciation to one another, and engage in activities that elicit positive emotions and a sense of connection.

4. Make quality time together a priority: Set aside intentional time to spend together without distractions. Setting aside date evenings,

organizing activities that you both enjoy, or simply having meaningful talks can all contribute to this.

5. Work on physical intimacy: Focus on repairing physical connection by exploring new physical methods to connect, both sexually and non-sexually. Non-sexual touch, such as holding hands, snuggling, or giving massages, is acceptable. Communicate your desires and boundaries in an open and honest

manner, and be willing to try new things together.

6. Seek professional help if necessary: If you're having trouble rebuilding intimacy on your own, consider couples therapy or counseling. A qualified therapist can help you reconnect on a deeper level by providing direction, facilitating good talks, and offering skills and approaches.

7. Show empathy and forgiveness: Recognize that both spouses may have contributed to the breakdown of closeness. Try to comprehend each other's experiences and viewpoints to practice empathy. Be empathetic to one another and strive to forgive previous wrongs or faults.

8. Patience and persistence: It takes time and effort to rebuild intimacy. It is important to be gentle with yourself and also with one another.

Recognize that improvement may take time and that setbacks are a normal part of the process. Continue conversing, expressing love and affection, and attempting to restore the emotional and physical connection.

Have it at the back of your mind that every relationship or union is different, and often times, what works for one couple may eventually not work for another. It's critical to tailor these stages to your personal relationship dynamics and demands. It is possible to reestablish and strengthen closeness in your relationship with commitment and a desire to put in the effort.

Rebuilding intimacy is a journey that involves both couples' dedication, patience, and work. This process must be approached with an open mind and a willingness to adapt and grow together. You also need to understand that every relationship is different like i earlier said, and there is no one particular way out. What works for one couple may not work for another, therefore it is critical to develop solutions that are tailored to your relationship's unique requirements and dynamics.

Finally, restoring closeness is achievable with commitment and a deliberate attempt to reconnect on emotional and physical levels.

Couples can reestablish the profound emotional and physical relationship that brought them together by addressing underlying issues, enhancing communication, promoting empathy, prioritizing physical connection, and getting professional treatment when necessary. Remember that intimacy is a journey that demands regular care and nurturing rather than a goal. Couples can heal and enhance their connection with patience, understanding, and love, leading to a more rewarding and intimate relationship.

CHAPTER 7: SETTING BOUNDARIES AND TRANSPARENCY: GUIDELINES FOR REBUILDING RELATIONSHIP TRUST

Any healthy and successful relationship is built on trust. When trust is destroyed, whether via infidelity, concealment, or other forms of betrayal, the relationship suffers and both partners feel hurt and vulnerable. Rebuilding trust takes time, effort, and a commitment to setting clear limits and encouraging transparency. In this post, we will address the significance of boundaries and transparency, as well as how to establish standards for regaining trust in a relationship.

1. Recognizing Boundaries:

Setting boundaries is critical in any relationship, but especially so when trust has been violated. Boundaries are the standards and boundaries we set to protect our mental and physical health. They serve as a framework for behavior, defining what is and is not acceptable. When trust is lost, boundaries can assist to create a sense of safety and set expectations to prevent additional harm.

2. Transparent Communication:

Transparency and open communication are inextricably intertwined. Rebuilding trust necessitates both couples openly sharing their feelings, worries, and relationship goals. It is critical to create an environment in which both individuals feel safe expressing themselves without fear of judgment or criticism. Encourage regular check-ins and set aside specific periods to discuss progress and issues.

3. Establishing Ground Rules:

It is critical to set clear ground rules for behaviors, actions, and expectations in order to regain confidence. After open and honest discussions, both spouses should agree on these norms. For example, if trust has been destroyed due to adultery, both parties may elect to implement a transparency rule, such as sharing location information or being accountable for their whereabouts. These ground rules promote consistency and aid in the rebuilding of trust by providing reassurance and accountability.

4. Forgiveness and patience:

Rebuilding trust takes time and requires both couples to be patient. It is critical to keep in mind that trust cannot be rebuilt immediately. It takes time for both the betrayed partner and the betrayer to establish their sincerity and determination to reform. Throughout this process, patience and understanding are essential. Furthermore, forgiving is essential in restoring trust. Forgiveness does not imply forgetting or accepting the actions that violated trust, but rather letting go of the rage and suffering caused by the betrayal.

5. Reliability and consistency:

Rebuilding trust requires consistency and dependability. It is critical to follow through on promises, pledges, and adjustments in order to show the betrayed spouse that the rebuilding process is taken seriously. To demonstrate commitment and generate confidence that the patterns that led to the betrayal will not be repeated, actions should match words. Consistency steadily builds trust, and the betrayed partner will begin to feel more comfortable and less apprehensive over time.

6. Seek Professional Assistance If Necessary:

Rebuilding trust can be a difficult and complicated task. Seeking professional support can be quite beneficial if both spouses are struggling to navigate the healing and rebuilding road. A qualified therapist can offer advice, resources, and methods, as well as enable open and honest discussion in a secure setting. Therapy can also assist reveal underlying issues that contributed to the breach of trust and provide effective solutions to them.

To summarize, trust is the foundation of any good relationship, and rebuilding it necessitates a commitment to setting clear limits and promoting transparency. Open communication, establishing ground rules, exercising patience and forgiveness, consistency, and dependability are all critical components in reestablishing trust. If necessary, seek professional assistance, since working with a therapist can provide further support and advice. Rebuilding trust takes time and effort from both partners, but it is possible to rebuild trust and

create a stronger, more resilient

relationship with dedication and a

shared commitment.

CHAPTER 8: SEEKING PROFESSIONAL ASSISTANCE: THE ROLE OF THERAPY IN RECOVERY FROM INFIDELITY

Infidelity in a relationship can cause enormous sorrow, betrayal, and upheaval. Discovering that one's partner has been unfaithful is a traumatic experience that can damage both parties. Recovering from such an emotional blow is difficult, but obtaining expert support via therapy may be extremely beneficial in healing and regaining trust. In this article, we will look at the various components of therapy in the context of infidelity, such as the benefits, tactics, and strategies used by therapists to help people heal.

Understanding Infidelity:

Infidelity refers to a variety of behaviors that violate the trust established between partners, including emotional, physical, and cyber affairs. It frequently results in broken self-esteem, overwhelming emotions, and a lack of faith in the partnership. Understanding the complexities of why infidelity occurs is critical for facilitating effective therapy sessions.

The Function of Therapy:

1. Creating a safe setting: Therapy creates a confidential and nonjudgmental environment in which individuals can communicate their feelings, anxieties, and thoughts

without fear of criticism or retaliation. Creating a sense of safety is critical for managing the stormy emotions that accompany infidelity.

2. Emotional processing: Infidelity sets off a chain reaction of feelings such as rage, despair, perplexity, and contempt. Individuals can get a better knowledge of their feelings and reactions through therapy, which helps them process and navigate these emotions. Individuals can begin

to recover and move forward by examining these feelings in a guided therapeutic context.

3. Rebuilding trust: Infidelity shatters trust, which is the foundation of any partnership. Therapy seeks to restore trust by addressing the underlying issues that led to the infidelity and developing new communication and transparency habits. Couples are guided through trust-building exercises by therapists, allowing

them to develop a strong foundation for their relationship.

4. Communication and conflict resolution: Infidelity is frequently the result of poor communication and unresolved problems. Couples can enhance their communication skills through therapy, allowing them to express themselves honestly and productively. Therapists educate couples healthy conflict resolution skills through guided conversations

and activities, boosting good communication and reducing future misunderstandings.

5. Addressing underlying issues: Infidelity can be a symptom of deeper issues in a relationship, such as a lack of intimacy, unresolved traumas, or unfulfilled needs. Therapy investigates these underlying difficulties, assisting individuals in gaining understanding of themselves and their interpersonal dynamics.

Individuals can strive towards mending and preventing future occurrences of infidelity by addressing these core reasons.

Methods of Infidelity Therapy:

1. Cognitive-Behavioral Therapy (CBT): Cognitive-Behavioral Therapy (CBT) focuses on recognizing and challenging negative beliefs and behaviors connected with infidelity. Therapists assist people in reframing their ideas and developing healthy

coping methods. This method can help reduce feelings of guilt, humiliation, and self-blame.

2. Emotionally Focused Therapy (EFT): EFT is a type of psychotherapy that focuses on understanding and changing the emotional dynamics of a relationship. Couples' attachment styles and emotional needs are explored by therapists, allowing for a greater connection and understanding. EFT can help with

healing by encouraging empathy, compassion, and emotional security.

3. Individual Therapy: Individual therapy allows each partner to explore their own personal experiences and feelings related to infidelity. Individuals can get insight into themselves, work on self-growth, and process their feelings autonomously using this strategy. Individual therapy can be especially

helpful when one partner is unwilling to participate in couples' therapy.

4. Group Therapy: Group therapy allows those who have suffered infidelity to interact, share their stories, and offer support to one another. Group therapy can offer a sense of belonging and validation. It enables people to recognize that they are not alone in their challenges and that they may benefit from the experiences of others.

Healing Techniques for Infidelity:

1. Recognizing and expressing feelings: Encouraging open and honest conversations about the spectrum of emotions felt, such as anger, sadness, and betrayal, is an important step towards healing. Therapists support these discussions and advise on healthy methods to express emotions.

2. Rebuilding trust: It takes time, commitment, and work from both

spouses to rebuild trust after infidelity. Therapy assists couples in establishing clear boundaries, developing new expectations, and working towards trust restoration. Couples are guided via exercises like as transparency, accountability, and consistent communication by therapists.

3. Improving communication skills: Improving communication skills is critical in mending a relationship

damaged by infidelity. Couples can benefit from therapy by learning new communication skills such as active listening, assertiveness, and empathy. Couples can use these abilities to express themselves effectively, acknowledge each other's emotions, and negotiate problems productively.

4. Improving intimacy: Infidelity frequently erodes connection in a partnership. Through activities that

create connection, intimacy building exercises, and reestablishing common interests, therapy focuses on helping couples rebuild emotional and physical closeness.

5. Forgiveness and reconciliation: Individuals may opt to explore forgiveness in therapy since it is a profoundly personal and complex process. Therapists conduct forgiveness sessions, assisting couples in exploring their own values,

beliefs, and capacity for forgiveness.

If reconciliation is wanted, it entails rebuilding the relationship on the basis of trust, honesty, and ongoing effort.

Conclusion

Infidelity healing is a difficult and nuanced process that takes patience, commitment, and professional help. Therapy is an important part of this journey because it provides a safe environment for people to process their feelings, address underlying issues, reestablish trust, and discover healthier ways of communicating. Couples and individuals can traverse the complex route to healing, growth, and the prospect of a renewed and stronger connection by using a variety of therapy approaches and strategies.

Seeking professional assistance is not a show of weakness, but rather a proactive move towards healing and rebuilding following infidelity. Individuals who engage in therapy can develop the tools and insights they need to negotiate their emotions, restore trust, and foster healthy communication and relationships. Couples can work with a qualified therapist to build a new, more robust relationship based on trust, understanding, and mutual respect.

Infidelity can be devastating to a relationship, but it does not have to be the end of the road. Couples can engage on a journey of healing, progress, and eventual restoration with expert assistance. Therapy can help people and couples rebuild trust, address underlying issues, improve communication skills, and establish a stronger, more satisfying relationship as they traverse the great sorrow and hardships of infidelity. Seeking professional help is a brave step

towards healing that should be

accepted as a crucial element of the

road to recovery and regeneration.

CHAPTER 9: MOVING FORWARD: STARTING OVER AFTER INFIDELITY

Infidelity is a terrible betrayal that is frequently regarded as a serious blow to the trust and basis of any partnership. However, following such an occurrence, it is possible to move on and develop a stronger, more resilient bond. This article will go over the actions to take in order to start again after infidelity, emphasizing open communication, professional help, personal growth, forgiveness, and trust restoration. Couples can engage on a recovery journey by identifying and treating the grief created by infidelity, ultimately cultivating a better and more rewarding relationship.

Understanding the Consequences of Infidelity

Infidelity can have a substantial influence on both couples' mental well-being. Anger, anguish, remorse, embarrassment, and perplexity are all common reactions to betrayal. The instant reaction may be to blame oneself, question one's self-worth, or become enraged at the unfaithful partner. It is critical to understand that these reactions are typical. Before beginning the healing process together, both couples should give themselves time to process these emotions on their own.

Communication that is open

Once the first emotions have been acknowledged and managed, both couples must openly share their feelings and opinions concerning the infidelity. The loyal partner must communicate their anguish, anger, and sadness, whilst the unfaithful partner must accept responsibility for their acts, apologize, and display a real desire to reestablish trust. Active listening, empathy, and a willingness to comprehend each other's perspectives without passing judgment are all components of open communication.

Professional Advice

Seeking expert assistance, such as couples therapy or relationship counseling, can be quite helpful in navigating the intricacies of reconstructing a relationship following infidelity. A competent therapist can give an objective space for both spouses to express their thoughts, work through challenges, and find healthier ways of interacting to one another. Couples can also be guided by therapists through the process of rebuilding trust, addressing underlying difficulties, and creating new communication habits.

Personal Development

As part of building a new beginning after infidelity, both partners must commit to personal growth and self-reflection. Individual therapy is used to address any underlying personal issues that may have contributed to the infidelity, such as low self-esteem, unresolved trauma, or unmet needs. Each partner can build a deeper sense of self and understand their own triggers by working on personal growth, allowing them to make healthier choices in their relationship.

Forgiveness

Moving forward after adultery necessitates forgiveness. Forgiveness, on the other hand, is a process that requires time and effort from both spouses. It does not imply ignoring or condoning the adultery, but rather letting go of the resentment and anger that can stymie the healing process. The loyal partner must be willing to forgive and let go of the grief created by infidelity, while the unfaithful partner must be patient and understanding, enabling the forgiveness process to evolve naturally. It is critical to understand that forgiveness does not always imply reconciliation. Each partner must make a unique decision depending on their circumstances and abilities to regain trust.

Restoring Trust

Rebuilding trust is a critical component of starting again after infidelity. It necessitates persistent effort, transparency, and honesty on the part of the unfaithful partner. The unfaithful partner must be willing to disclose the infidelity fully, answer all questions honestly, and accept responsibility for their conduct. Trust is rebuilt via constant activities such as dependability, honoring promises, and keeping channels of communication open. The faithful partner should also actively participate in repairing trust by being open to healing and providing opportunities for the unfaithful partner to reestablish trust over time.

Setting Boundaries and Commitment

To avoid future breaches of trust, it is critical to establish clear limits and obligations following infidelity. Both partners should freely address their expectations and establish mutually agreed-upon communication, transparency, and fidelity boundaries. Sharing passwords, having unrestricted access to electronic devices, limiting interactions with members of the opposite sex, or arranging regular check-ins to discuss any concerns or triggers are all examples of boundaries. Both partners must understand and respect these boundaries in order to rebuild trust and sustain a healthy relationship.

Relationship Maintenance

Making a new start after infidelity necessitates a commitment to nurture the relationship. Prioritizing quality time together, engaging in activities that deepen the emotional connection, and constantly working on effective communication skills are all part of this. Regular date nights, weekend trips, or participating in common activities can help remind both couples of their love and connection. Furthermore, regular communication regarding the healing process's progress and resolving any concerns that may occur along the way is critical in sustaining the connection and preventing future disagreements.

Although infidelity can be heartbreaking in any relationship, it is possible to start over and reestablish trust and love. Open communication, seeking professional advice, personal growth, forgiveness, and establishing limits and commitments are all critical aspects in the healing process. Both partners can go on and develop a stronger, more robust bond marked by trust, understanding, and a renewed sense of commitment by actively working on these characteristics. It is critical to remember that rebuilding a relationship after infidelity requires time, patience, and work on the side of both spouses. However, with a real desire for healing and progress, a new and rewarding future can be created together.